How I Survived 40 Years With Diabetes

by

Marek Woźniak

Copyright © 2024 Marek Woźniak

All rights reserved.

DISCLAIMER

The material in this book is intended primarily for general informational purposes; it should not be used in place of professional medical advice, diagnosis, or treatment.

Always consult your physician or other qualified healthcare provider if you have any questions about diabetes or any other medical matter. Never ignore or delay medical advice from a professional because of something you have read in this book. Any health problems resulting from the use or misuse of the materials in this book are not the responsibility of the author or publisher.

You assume full responsibility for any reliance you place on the information contained in this book. Because the medical field is constantly changing, new information may become available that will affect the accuracy of the content. Contact your physician immediately if you think you may have a medical problem. This book does not recommend self-diagnosis or self-treatment. It is essential that you speak with your healthcare provider before making any decisions about your health.

TABLE OF CONTENTS

Introduction 5

Day One – Why Me? 6

Diabetes Doesn't Close Doors 9

Rules and Your New Habits 11

Understanding Insulin Action 14

Strategies to Stop and Think Twice 16

Attitude – The Fight in My Mind 20

Strategies to Strengthen Your Mental Resolve 22

Activity Development – Mental Fitness 23

Traveling with Diabetes 26

Physical Activity and Mental Fitness 28

Adopting New Rules and Habits 29

Have to Know Your Body 30

Dawn Phenomenon and the Somogyi Effect 33

Me and the Outside World – How We Are Perceived 35

Daily Habits and Emotional Well-Being 37

Dealing with Diabetes Burnout 39

Daily Habits and Long-Term Success 41

References 42

ABOUT THE AUTHOR 44

Introduction

Every illness determines what kind of man you are. Diabetes made me realize how important consistency is and that my mental toughness was just as important to my survival as my physical health. How we approach everyday obstacles, particularly those associated with illness, is shaped by our mentality. The struggle frequently occurs in our mind, where our ideas have the potential to either encourage us to follow the rules or deter us from doing so.

When I found out I had diabetes at 19, it felt like everything had changed. I was a young, energetic, future-oriented person. But the diagnosis was a sobering reminder that I was just dust in the wind.

Day One – Why Me?

I felt awful and scared of injections. But after a few hours in the hospital and a couple of injections, everything seemed normal again—or so I thought. Could I go back to my old life? Unfortunately, no. Instead, I was handed a few yellowed guides about healthy eating, exercise, and controlling blood sugar levels. It all seemed like a mistake—I was a student! I didn't have time for this. I had exams to prepare for.

That was the beginning of an emotional rollercoaster. My story was just getting started.

Hearing the words "You have diabetes" feels like being hit by a tidal wave.But accepting these feelings is a key part of the process.

Acceptance doesn't mean giving up. It means recognizing that diabetes is now a part of your life and that you can move forward by focusing on what you can control. Establish a routine that includes balanced meals, exercise, and stress management. These habits will form the backbone of your diabetes management plan, helping you find balance in your daily life.

Over time, mental strength takes root. It doesn't happen overnight, but consistent action helps reduce insecurities and builds confidence. This journey will test your resilience, but it will also show you how strong you really are.

The first day of your diabetes journey is not only a

challenge, but it will also change the way you view life. Every difficult situation brings with it a lesson, and for me, it opened my eyes to things I hadn't considered before.

Acceptance doesn't mean giving up. It means recognizing that diabetes is now a part of your life and that you can move forward by focusing on what you can control. Establish a routine that includes balanced meals, exercise, and stress management. These habits will form the backbone of your diabetes management plan, helping you find balance in your daily life.

Over time, mental strength takes root. It doesn't happen overnight, but consistent action helps reduce insecurities and builds confidence. This journey will test your resilience, but it will also show you how strong you really are.

The first day of your diabetes journey is not only a challenge, but also a change in the way you view life. Every difficult situation brings with it a lesson, and for me, it opened my eyes to things I hadn't considered before. I realized how vital family support was and how every day truly mattered. The disease humbled me and taught me to be grateful for what I have.

You must live your life as normally as possible, just like anyone else would.

I've always tried to follow this principle. I never made a big deal out of my illness. Whether I was traveling, working, or at a party, I did my best to manage things quietly. In time, others began treating me that way too. Of course, there were times when I went to events and there was nothing for me to eat—fatty food and sugary drinks everywhere. Or I'd get the usual questions: "Why aren't you eating?" Sometimes I delayed taking my insulin because work felt more urgent.In retrospect, I see that this was a mistake.

It is important to live a "normal" life, but it is equally important to follow the rules. It took me a long time to feel comfortable giving myself injections in public places, such as restaurants or parties, without worrying about what people would think. The biggest mistake I made was allowing others to influence me and break my own health rules.

One of the hardest things to face with diabetes is thinking about what you may never do or enjoy again. Favorite foods, spontaneous adventures, even career goals can seem out of reach. We often mourn the life we imagined we'd have and worry about the limits diabetes imposes.

Diabetes Doesn't Close Doors

I met people who trained intensely in weightlifting, a girl who ran marathons, and people who raced MTB. Even several presidents had diabetes.

Dealing with diabetes doesn't mean giving up on your dreams. There are so many well-known and respected people with diabetes who have not only survived, but thrived, using their platforms to inspire others. Their stories are proof that diabetes doesn't have to get in the way of a fulfilling life.

Academy Award-winning actress Halle Berry was diagnosed with type 1 diabetes at age 22. Despite that, she has built an incredibly successful acting career, known for her roles in Monster's Ball and X-Men. She openly shares her story, emphasizing the importance of a healthy diet and exercise. In addition to being an actress, Halle is also a diabetes advocate, helping to raise awareness and support others.

Renowned and respected actor Tom Hanks was diagnosed with type 2 diabetes later in life. He continues to give Oscar-winning performances and reflects on the role his lifestyle played in his diagnosis. Hanks' openness has sparked important conversations about type 2 diabetes and the lifestyle changes needed to manage the disease.

Nick Jonas, who was diagnosed with type 1 diabetes at just 13, used his diagnosis as motivation to pursue his dreams. Today, he's not only a global pop star, but also co-founder of the Beyond Type 1 Foundation, which raises awareness and funds diabetes research.

Former NFL quarterback Jay Cutler is one of the athletes that demonstrate that diabetes need not prevent an athlete from pursuing their athletic profession. Even after receiving a Type 1 diabetes diagnosis throughout his football career, Cutler was still able to lead a healthy lifestyle and play at the top of his game.

Additionally, well-known singer Patti LaBelle had a Type 2 diabetes diagnosis in the 1990s. Following the shock of learning she had diabetes, she published a cookbook and changed her lifestyle. She uses her voice to spread awareness of diabetes in addition to singing. These pictures demonstrate that diabetes is a fight that can be won with the correct mindset, encouragement, and commitment to self-care. There is more to it than that.

Rules and Your New Habits

As we get older, our memory naturally declines—it's part of the aging process, not just diabetes. There have been countless times when I've either forgotten to take my insulin or accidentally taken it twice because I couldn't remember. To solve this, I developed a simple system. Depending on when I take my insulin—whether it's morning, afternoon, or evening—I place the container differently each time. For example, after my morning injection, I place the insulin box on its large side, and after my pre-dinner injection, I place it on the small side.

I've found that having this small practice has made it easier for me to remember my insulin dosages. The secret to effectively treating diabetes is to establish a regular regimen. Blood sugar levels may be kept extremely steady with the use of regular meal timings, medication regimens, and physical exercise.

Starting your day by checking your blood sugar and logging your meals and activities can provide valuable information. Even better is continuous blood sugar monitoring. These devices measure your blood sugar every minute and send a reading to your smartphone.

Additionally, they alert you when your levels are too high or low. My diabetes has stabilized since I started using one of these devices. You can see trends and adjust your treatment strategy as needed with the help of this regular practice.

Consistency is what stabilizes blood sugar levels. Setting

reminders on your phone for medication and meals can help me avoid any disruptions in your schedule. Building these habits into your daily routine makes it easier to anticipate and prevent blood sugar spikes or drops.

Special events, such as family gatherings or work events, require careful planning. I always carry a diabetes kit with me, which includes my medications, a blood glucose monitor, and a few quick-acting sources of glucose, such as glucose tablets or juice. If I'm attending an event with an unfamiliar menu, I try to eat a small, balanced meal beforehand to make sure I don't overindulge. Planning ahead makes it easier to avoid temptation and helps me stay on track with my blood sugar goals.

When I go to parties, I also make sure to enquire about the menu in advance and, if needed, bring a meal that I know will work for my diabetes. I can eat in this way without worrying about my blood sugar levels. My usual choices include veggies, whole grains, and lean meats; I stay away from items that are heavy in sugar or carbohydrates.

If alcohol is served, I limit it and choose lower-sugar options.

Cravings are inevitable, especially in social settings where tempting foods are everywhere.

focusing on moderation and careful eating is the key. Be mindful of your hunger and satiety cues, savor every taste, and pay attention to what you're eating. I've also discovered that keeping wholesome snacks like almonds, apples, or yogurt on hand helps me resist the need to overindulge. I remind myself of the drawbacks of consuming a lot of sugar or carbs and choose for healthier alternatives. It's beneficial to have a reliable and trustworthy person. You may encourage others to accept your choices by being open about your dietary restrictions.

Understanding Insulin Action

To effectively manage diabetes, understanding how insulin works in your body is crucial. Insulin therapy is not a one-size-fits-all solution—it depends on the type of insulin you use, your lifestyle, and how your body responds to it.

Insulin action refers to how soon insulin begins to lower your blood sugar after injection. This timing is critical to managing blood sugar spikes, especially around meals. *Duration* refers to how long the insulin continues working in your body. Knowing both the action and duration of your insulin is essential for managing blood sugar throughout the day.

Ideally, insulin should match the rate at which your blood sugar rises after a meal. But even with modern insulin options, perfect synchronization can be difficult, especially if you're eating high-glycemic index (GI) foods. These foods can cause a rapid spike in blood sugar, making it harder for insulin to keep up.

Carbohydrate counting plays a huge role in managing insulin doses effectively. By understanding the number of carbs in your meals, you can better predict how much insulin you'll need to cover them. The American Diabetes Association (ADA) recommends keeping carb intake consistent at each meal to avoid spikes or drops in blood sugar. Common sources of carbohydrates include fruits, vegetables, grains, and dairy.

But managing diabetes isn't just about counting carbs.

Eating a *balanced diet*—one that includes lean proteins, healthy fats, and whole grains—can help keep blood sugar stable. Limiting processed foods, sugary drinks, and high-fat meals can further prevent sudden blood sugar spikes and support overall health.

Strategies to Stop and Think Twice

One evening I spontaneously decided to go to the cinema with friends. In the rush of excitement I forgot about my planned insulin injection. Sitting in the cinema I could feel my blood sugar rising and there was nothing I could do about it.

In hindsight, I know I should have said, "Sorry, I can go with you, but I need to handle something first."

One of the most valuable lessons diabetes has taught me is the importance of stopping and thinking twice about my choices—especially when it comes to food. Seemingly small decisions can have major consequences. It's essential to understand this and make careful choices to effectively manage diabetes.

Imagine you're at a family gathering, a holiday party, or just out with friends. The table is full of tempting treats—cookies, cakes, and sugary drinks.

Everyone else is having a good time, and someone says, "Just eat one bite! It won't hurt!" It's a scenario that many of us with diabetes often face. The pressure to join in is immense, but we know that these situations require a different approach.

Consuming meals heavy in sugar or carbs can cause fast rises in blood sugar levels in diabetics, which can cause unpleasant symptoms including increased thirst, weariness, and frequent urination. More significantly, recurrent surges may lead to long-term issues such harm to the kidneys, heart, nerves, eyes, and kidneys.

Giving in to temptation on a regular basis can result in poor blood sugar control over time. This increases the risk of developing serious complications like cardiovascular disease, neuropathy, retinopathy, and kidney failure. It's not just about that one bite—it's about the cumulative effect of your choices over the months and years.

Here's how to go:

Plan ahead: Eat a healthy meal that includes protein, fiber, and healthy fats before going to an event that has tempting foods. Eat only what's good for you at the event and don't worry about what others think.

Educate your friends and family: Help your loved ones understand the impact diabetes has on your life. Once they know, they'll be more likely to support your choices and less likely to pressure you into eating something unhealthy.

Bring your own alternatives: If you're going to an event, bring a diabetes-friendly snack that you can enjoy. This way, you won't feel left out and can still indulge in something sweet without compromising your health.

Practice Mindfulness: Before you eat, pause and think about how the food will affect your blood sugar and your long-term health. Consider the emotional and physical consequences of your choices.

Stay Committed to Your Health Goals: Remind yourself

why you're making these choices. Your long-term health and well-being are worth the short-term sacrifice of skipping that treat.

Living with diabetes means practicing constant vigilance and thoughtful decision-making. It's not about depriving yourself—it's about making choices that support your health and well-being. By using a stop-and-think strategy, you can navigate social situations and temptations with confidence and grace. Every choice you make is a step toward a healthier future.

One of the basic pieces of information regarding food selection is the glycemic index (GI). The Glycemic Index (GI) measures how quickly carbohydrate-containing foods raise your blood sugar levels. Foods are ranked on a scale from 0 to 100, with pure glucose being assigned a value of 100.

- Low-GI foods (55 or less) are absorbed more slowly, leading to a gradual rise in blood sugar. Examples include whole grains, legumes, and most fruits and vegetables.

- Medium-GI foods (56-69) include items like whole wheat bread and sweet potatoes.

- High-GI foods (70 and above) include white bread, sugary snacks, and rice.

Using the GI to guide your food choices helps you maintain stable blood sugar levels throughout the day. For instance, pairing high-GI foods with low-GI foods in a meal can moderate the overall impact on your blood sugar. A practical example is pairing white rice with beans and vegetables to lower the meal's overall GI, which helps prevent sharp spikes.

By incorporating the GI into your diabetes management plan, you can make smarter food choices that lead to more consistent blood sugar control, improved energy levels, and overall better health.

Attitude – The Fight in My Mind

Being optimistic does not imply denying the reality of having diabetes. It entails facing such facts with an attitude that prioritizes finding answers above creating difficulties. It all comes down to having the belief that you can control your situation and acting on that belief. Your mental outlook plays a huge role in your physical health—it influences your willingness to stick to a healthy diet, exercise regularly, and monitor your blood sugar.

But maintaining a positive attitude isn't always easy. There will be times when you feel restricted by the lifestyle changes diabetes requires. Whether it's the urge to eat a forbidden food or the temptation to skip a workout, the battle is often internal - it's inside your head.

Consider an instance in the past when you felt obliged to break the rules. A sweet treat could have appeared like a comforting diversion on an especially stressful day.Or maybe you didn't want to stand out from the crowd at a party.These scenarios try your determination and bring to light the psychological difficulties associated with treating diabetes.

Even while giving in might occasionally appear innocent, there are actual consequences. Your blood sugar may rise and then fall after eating this delicacy, leaving you feeling both invigorated and worn out. Repeatedly breaking the guidelines can eventually result in poor blood sugar management, which raises the risk of long-term issues.

In addition, breaking the rules can start a vicious cycle.

You destroy your self-esteem and make it harder to continue on your current course every time you give up. For this reason, it is crucial to win the mental war by creating coping mechanisms that keep you in a good mood.

Strategies to Strengthen Your Mental Resolve

Create achievable goals: Break down your long-term health goals into smaller, more manageable tasks. To stay motivated, celebrate the small wins you have along the way.

Remind yourself to be kind to yourself: No one is perfect, and failures happen. Reflect on what led to your mistakes and how to prevent them from happening again, rather than punishing yourself for making them.

Visualize success: Spend a few minutes each day visualizing yourself successfully managing your diabetes. Imagine the positive results of sticking to your health plan—feeling energized and avoiding complications.

Remain educated: Making educated decisions will be simpler the more you know about the management of diabetes. Confidence comes from knowledge.

Create a network of support: Get close to people who are aware of your struggles and are rooting for you. This might be a support group for diabetics, medical professionals, friends, or family.

Every day is a struggle to maintain optimism and withstand temptation. You may more successfully manage your diabetes and lead a happier, more satisfying life by strengthening your resilience and concentrating on your health objectives.

Activity Development – Mental Fitness

Even though I'm not the most physically active person, I always find ways to incorporate movement into my daily routine. I enjoy biking, hiking, and swimming when I can. But even in my daily routine, I make small changes to stay active. To walk an additional mile, for instance, I park my car approximately 1,000 steps away from my place of employment. I use the stairs instead of the elevator when I'm at work. In this manner, I am able to complete around 5,000–7,000 steps.

Diabetes is not just a physical condition — it's a complex lifestyle challenge that requires a balance of physical activity and mental fitness. After living with diabetes for more than four decades, I've learned that staying physically active while constantly improving your mental fitness is key to thriving, not just surviving.

Keeping up an active lifestyle is crucial for diabetes management. As per the American Diabetes Association (ADA), engaging in regular exercise improves blood sugar regulation, boosts general physical health, and lowers the likelihood of cardiovascular ailments. Easy exercises like swimming, cycling, or walking can greatly increase the body's sensitivity to insulin, facilitating a more effective utilization of glucose by the body.

But just as important as physical activity is mental fitness. Keeping your mind sharp helps you manage the daily challenges of diabetes—whether it's making decisions about your diet, managing medications, or problem-solving on the fly. Engaging in memory training exercises, puzzles, or brain games keeps the mind healthy and sharp. Research has indicated that cognitive training might enhance mental performance in senior citizens, particularly beneficial for people with conditions like diabetes that necessitate continuous vigilance. One of the greatest things I could do to keep my mind active was to play an instrument. Research indicates that musical training can enhance cognitive abilities, improve memory, and boost emotional well-being. Learning to play the guitar has brought me a lot of joy, relieved stress, and sharpened my cognitive abilities.

Social interaction also plays a big role in maintaining mental fitness. Isolation and loneliness can have a negative effect on diabetes management, making it harder to stick to a health routine. I've made an effort to stay connected with friends and family, join diabetes support groups, and participate in community events. I feel like I belong and receive emotional support and helpful counsel from these social ties.

Reading seems to do a very good job of keeping my mind active. Read everything from fiction to self-help books to IT classes pertinent to my field of work; reading enhances cognitive function, reduces stress, and postpones cognitive decline. Reading has helped me learn and acquire knowledge that has enhanced my capacity to manage my illness.

Maintaining a busy career has also been essential to my mental health. My work in IT has given me a feeling of purpose and intellectual stimulation. I'm always seeking opportunities for professional development, attending workshops, and learning new skills related to my field.

Education has been particularly important in managing my diabetes. I've kept myself informed about the latest research, treatments, and dietary recommendations. Resources like the ADA website, medical journals, and diabetes education programs have been invaluable. My ability to make wise decisions and take charge of my diabetes management increased as I gained more knowledge about my illness. The two main pillars of my diabetes journey have been emotional and physical health. Exercises that mix mindfulness with physical movement, such as yoga and tai chi, have been shown to be very effective in lowering stress, enhancing mental clarity, and increasing flexibility.

By incorporating a variety of activities, from physical exercise and mental training to socializing and continuous learning, you can lead a fulfilling and healthy life with diabetes. Embrace these practices, stay informed, and maintain a positive mindset. Both your body and mind will benefit from the effort.

Traveling with Diabetes

When you have diabetes, traveling might be difficult, but with good planning, you can enjoy your trip without any issues. I make care to look up the availability of pharmacies and medical services in my location before I go. Keeping all my diabetes supplies in my carry-on luggage ensures they won't be lost or damaged during transit.

Another important step is wearing a medical ID bracelet and carrying a doctor's note that explains my condition and the medications I'm using. This can be helpful in case of any medical emergencies or security checks, especially when flying.

Planning meals and snacks ahead of time is also critical.

It's also a good idea to take snacks like fruits, nuts, or low-sugar protein bars to help stabilize blood sugar while on the run.

Moving west will effectively extend your day, therefore you may need to adjust your insulin dosage. The American Diabetes Association (ADA) suggests that in order to make up for the longer day, you would need to eat more meals and potentially even take an extra dose of insulin. Speak with your healthcare provider to make sure your long-acting insulin dose is adjusted while traveling between time zones.

Traveling east shortens the day, so you may need to skip a meal or adjust your insulin dose to prevent hypoglycemia.

How I survived 40 years with diabetes

The ADA suggests monitoring your blood sugar more frequently on travel days and bringing extra snacks to deal with unexpected drops in blood sugar.

Both cases require regular blood sugar checks and maintaining a healthy fluid intake. Prepare your vacation ahead of time by packing a thorough itinerary, additional supplies, and emergency contacts.

Those who with diabetes have some special difficulties when flying. During lengthy trips, blood sugar levels can be affected by time zone shifts, modified food plans, and insufficient physical exercise.

To manage this, I adjust my medication and meal schedule according to my destination's time zone.

Staying hydrated is particularly important during flights. I drink plenty of water and avoid alcohol and caffeine, which can cause dehydration. I also let the flight attendants know that I have diabetes, in case I need assistance during the flight.

On long flights, I attempt to take quick steps about the cabin to improve circulation and reduce the risk of blood clots. Additionally, since on-board meals may not always be diabetes-friendly, it's imperative to pack extra snacks. I can always manage my blood sugar levels when I have low-carb snacks on hand, even while I'm on the go.

Physical Activity and Mental Fitness

One of the best strategies to maintain stable blood sugar levels and enhance general health is through physical activity. Whether it's a daily bike ride, a yoga class, or a stroll, I try to fit fitness into my schedule whenever I can. I routinely monitor my blood sugar before and after doing out to see how my body responds. It's also crucial to have a snack with you while you exercise in case your blood sugar drops.

Frequent exercise improves mental health in addition to managing diabetes.

If you find hobbies that you like, like swimming or hiking, you're more likely to remain with it. It has been demonstrated that participating in a group workout program or class helps to maintain your motivation and accountability.

Mental and physical well-being are equally important for diabetes management.

Learning good coping mechanisms is important because stress and anxiety can affect blood sugar levels.

I've found that mindfulness, deep breathing, and meditation are great ways to manage stress. Talking to others has also been a huge help in dealing with the emotional elements of chronic illness, whether through professional therapy or diabetes support groups.

Adopting New Rules and Habits

Adopting new rules and habits has empowered me to manage diabetes effectively, allowing me to not just survive but thrive. By preparing for events, resisting temptation, planning for travel, and staying active, you can take control of your diabetes and lead a fulfilling life. Every small step toward better management is progress, and with dedication and perseverance, you can turn challenges into opportunities for growth and resilience.

Have to Know Your Body

One of the most crucial aspects of managing diabetes is truly knowing your body. Everyone with diabetes responds differently to factors like insulin, food, stress, and physical activity. Learning how your body reacts in different situations is essential for staying in control of your health.

For instance, I've learned that one unit of rapid-acting insulin lowers my blood sugar by about 30 mg/dL, but this isn't always exact. Several factors influence how well insulin works, including the type of meal I've eaten, my stress levels, physical activity, and even the timing of my injection. Drinking water can also help lower blood sugar, although the effect can vary depending on the situation.

One of the key things I've had to master is the timing of insulin injections relative to meals. Fast-acting insulin typically starts working 15-30 minutes after injection, which is crucial because blood sugar begins to rise about 10-15 minutes after eating. Synchronizing the timing of my insulin with the rise in blood sugar has been vital to managing post-meal spikes.

I've found that injecting insulin about 15 minutes before meals works best for me, but I always monitor my blood sugar and adjust based on the situation. If my blood sugar is low before a meal, I'll wait to inject insulin until after I eat. However, every person's response is unique, and these strategies should always be discussed with a healthcare provider before making adjustments.

How I survived 40 years with diabetes

Understanding the relationship between insulin requirements and blood sugar fluctuations has also been key. The lower your insulin needs, the fewer fluctuations you'll experience in blood sugar levels. Achieving stable, lower insulin doses requires consistent attention to diet, exercise, and stress management.

Carbohydrate counting has been another game-changer for me. By understanding the carbohydrate content in my meals and using that information to fine-tune my insulin dosage, I've been able to avoid significant highs and lows in blood sugar.

Physical exercise plays a crucial role as well. Exercise enhances insulin sensitivity and helps the body use glucose more efficiently. However, different types of exercise affect blood sugar levels differently. That's why I monitor my blood sugar before, during, and after exercise. This gives me a clear understanding of how my body reacts and allows me to make any necessary adjustments—like having a small snack before exercising to prevent hypoglycemia.

Stress and fatigue also have a big impact on blood sugar levels. When you're stressed, your body releases hormones like cortisol and adrenaline, which can raise blood sugar levels. Similarly, fatigue, often caused by poor sleep, can lead to insulin resistance, making it harder to control blood sugar.

Learning how to manage stress through techniques like meditation and yoga has helped me stabilize my blood sugar levels. Prioritizing sleep and maintaining a regular sleep schedule has also made a noticeable difference in how I feel and how well my body responds to insulin.

Dietary fats can further complicate blood sugar control by slowing down digestion. This often delays the rise in blood sugar, making it harder to predict when the insulin will start working. When I eat high-fat meals, I sometimes split my insulin dose or use a dual-wave bolus on my insulin pump to spread the insulin over a longer period of time. This helps me better manage delayed blood sugar spikes.

Knowing when and how much to eat something sweet is also critical for managing *hypoglycemia* (low blood sugar). The ADA recommends consuming 15-20 grams of fast-acting carbohydrates—like glucose tablets or juice—when your blood sugar drops below 70 mg/dL. I always keep glucose tablets or candy on hand, and after consuming a quick source of sugar, I recheck my blood sugar after 15 minutes to make sure it has risen to a safe level. It's important to avoid over-treating hypoglycemia, as this can cause blood sugar to swing too high.

Understanding your body is key to managing diabetes effectively. By paying attention to how your body responds to insulin, exercise, stress, and diet, you can achieve better control over your blood sugar levels and lead a healthier, more balanced life.

Dawn Phenomenon and the Somogyi Effect

One of the trickiest parts of managing diabetes for me has been dealing with the *Dawn Phenomenon*. For years, I struggled to control it, and even now, I sometimes see it affect me, even after a short nap during the day.

The Dawn Phenomenon happens when stress hormones like cortisol, glucagon, and adrenaline are released while you sleep. These hormones prompt your liver to release glucose into your bloodstream, causing your blood sugar levels to rise. For someone without diabetes, their body naturally produces more insulin to handle this glucose surge. However, for people with diabetes—especially if we don't take enough insulin at night—it can lead to high fasting blood sugar levels in the morning.

I've found that reducing my evening meal size and drinking more water before bed has helped me manage the Dawn Phenomenon more effectively. Hydration, in particular, always seems to make a difference for me. But like many things in diabetes management, what works for one person may not work for another. That's why it's so important to keep track of how your body responds and adjust your routine accordingly.

The *Somogyi Effect*, on the other hand, is different from the Dawn Phenomenon. It occurs when you experience low blood sugar (hypoglycemia) during the night, and your body overcompensates by releasing stress hormones that cause your blood sugar to spike by the time you wake up.

The difference between the Somogyi Effect and the Dawn Phenomenon is that the Somogyi Effect is preceded by an episode of hypoglycemia, whereas the Dawn Phenomenon is simply a rise in blood sugar levels in the early morning due to hormonal changes.

Both phenomena highlight the importance of monitoring your blood sugar levels, especially overnight. Understanding how your body reacts during sleep allows you to make necessary adjustments, whether it's through insulin dosage, meal timing, or hydration.

The best way to deal with these phenomena is with an insulin pump, which measures blood sugar and doses insulin automatically. Since I've been using CGM, I've learned how my body reacts. CGM was a game changer for me.

Me and the Outside World – How We Are Perceived

Since I started using continuous glucose monitoring (CGM), it has completely changed the way I manage my diabetes. Having the ability to check my blood sugar levels in real-time—on my phone, no less—has been a game-changer. With CGM, I can immediately see when my blood sugar is rising or dropping and take action quickly to correct it. It's been incredibly empowering.

However, using this technology in public sometimes changes how people perceive me. When others see me checking my phone in a restaurant or during a meeting, they might assume I'm just scrolling through social media. But once they realize I'm managing my diabetes, I often notice a shift in how they view me—they start to see me as a "sick" person.

People's perceptions of diabetes vary widely. I've experienced everything from sympathy and curiosity to misunderstanding and even unsolicited advice. Some people are genuinely interested and ask thoughtful questions about my condition, while others may view it through a lens of pity or misconception. I've also encountered people who feel the need to offer advice, even though they don't fully understand what it's like to live with diabetes.

One of the most challenging aspects of living with diabetes is how others interpret your behaviors. For example, after an insulin injection or meal, I sometimes wait before doing activities like driving, to ensure my blood sugar levels are stable. To people who don't know about diabetes, this can seem overly cautious or even neurotic. But in reality, it's an essential step to ensure my safety and health.

Every illness, including diabetes, changes you as a person. I often wonder how different my life would be if I didn't have diabetes, how it has shaped the person I am today, and how I would be if I were healthy. One thing I didn't fully understand when I was first diagnosed was the concept of *burnout*. It's something that happens repeatedly over the course of living with diabetes. It's easy to fall into a pattern where you stop measuring your blood sugar as frequently, skip meals, or become inconsistent with insulin. In those moments, everything starts to feel out of control.

When this happens, it's not just your health that suffers— your loved ones feel the impact too. I've experienced many moments where my lack of self-care affected the people closest to me. These are memories I'd rather forget, but they've taught me valuable lessons about managing my condition more thoughtfully.

Living with diabetes affects not only you but also the people around you. It's something I've learned to be mindful of, as my actions and health choices impact those I care about.

Daily Habits and Emotional Well-Being

Your daily habits significantly impact your ability to manage diabetes effectively. It's not just about insulin and diet—exercise, sleep, and stress management are equally important for maintaining balance and overall well-being.

Exercise is one of the most powerful tools for managing diabetes. Physical activity lowers blood sugar levels and improves insulin sensitivity, making it easier for your body to use glucose efficiently. The ADA recommends getting at least 150 minutes of moderate aerobic activity per week. Activities like walking, cycling, or swimming are great options. Just be sure to check your blood sugar before and after exercising to avoid hypoglycemia.

Sleep is another essential component of diabetes management. Poor sleep can disrupt insulin sensitivity, making blood sugar levels harder to control. Establishing a regular sleep routine and creating a restful sleep environment can help improve both sleep quality and blood sugar regulation. The Centers for Disease Control and Prevention (CDC) recommends getting 7 to 9 hours of sleep per night to support overall health.

Managing *stress* is also critical. When you're stressed, your body releases hormones like cortisol and adrenaline, which can raise blood sugar levels. Practicing relaxation techniques like deep breathing, meditation, or yoga can help manage stress and keep blood sugar levels stable. Support groups or counseling can also provide emotional support and practical advice for dealing with the mental challenges of diabetes.

Dealing with Diabetes Burnout

Living with diabetes day in and day out can wear anyone down. I first experienced *diabetes burnout* a few years after my diagnosis. At first, I followed my routine religiously—monitoring my blood sugar, taking medications, and maintaining a strict lifestyle. But after a while, the constant effort began to feel overwhelming. I wanted to break free from the routine of scheduled insulin injections and regular meals.

I began skipping blood sugar checks, neglecting my diet, and distancing myself from my health routine. Over time, I felt more and more isolated, and my motivation to manage my diabetes took a hit.

Burnout is something that happens to many people living with chronic illnesses, especially diabetes. It's that state of emotional and physical exhaustion where the daily demands of managing your condition feel like too much. For me, it manifested as frustration, anxiety, and a desire to just ignore it all.

But recognizing burnout early is key. If you can identify the signs before they take over, you can address the problem before it becomes too severe. Everyone's experienced that moment where you just want to take a break from it all, but when you have diabetes, it's important to find ways to push through that feeling without compromising your health.

Dealing with diabetes burnout is an ongoing process. It requires patience, self-compassion, and sometimes a change in your routine to prevent things from feeling monotonous. Seeking support from friends, family, or diabetes support groups can make a huge difference too. When you're struggling, it's essential to reach out and get the help you need.

While burnout is a natural part of living with diabetes, it doesn't have to derail your health management entirely. By recognizing the signs, making room for self-care, and staying flexible in your approach, you can work through it and continue managing your diabetes effectively.

Daily Habits and Long-Term Success

Daily habits are the backbone of successful diabetes management. Consistent exercise, balanced meals, regular sleep, and effective stress management are all part of the equation. It's also important to stay connected with your healthcare team, keep learning about new treatment options, and adjust your habits based on your body's needs.

When it comes to managing diabetes, there are no bad questions. Whether it's about the timing of insulin injections, how certain foods affect blood sugar, or navigating travel with diabetes, every question leads to a deeper understanding of how to manage the condition better.

Asking questions helps you learn more about your body, your needs, and how best to manage your blood sugar. The more you seek knowledge, the more confident and empowered you'll become in handling diabetes day by day.

The more you ask, the more you learn. Seeking knowledge and support is essential in staying confident and empowered on your diabetes journey. Every challenge you overcome adds to your resilience and ability to thrive with diabetes.

References

- American Diabetes Association. (2019). Diabetes and Mind/Body Connection. Retrieved from https://www.diabetes.org

- American Diabetes Association. (2020). Physical Activity/Exercise and Diabetes: A Position Statement of the American Diabetes Association. Diabetes Care, 29(6), 1433-1438.

- Ball, K., Berch, D. B., Helmers, K. F., et al. (2002). Effects of Cognitive Training Interventions With Older Adults: A Randomized Controlled Trial. JAMA, 288(18), 2271–2281.

- Hanna-Pladdy, B., & Mackay, A. (2011). The Relation Between Instrumental Musical Activity and Cognitive Aging. Neuropsychology, 25(3), 378–386.

- Luo, Y., Hawkley, L. C., Waite, L. J., & Cacioppo, J. T. (2012). Loneliness, Health, and Mortality in Old Age: A National Longitudinal Study. Social Science & Medicine, 74(6), 907-914.

- Neurology. (2013). Cognitive Activity and Cognitive Decline in Older Adults. 81(12), 986-991.

- American Diabetes Association. (2020). Standards of Medical Care in Diabetes—2020 Abridged for

Primary Care Providers. Clinical Diabetes, 38(1), 10-38.

- Colberg, S. R., Sigal, R. J., Yardley, J. E., et al. (2010). Physical Activity/Exercise and Diabetes: A Position Statement of the American Diabetes Association. Diabetes Care, 33(12), e147-e167.

- Lloyd, C., Smith, J., & Weinger, K. (2019). Stress and Diabetes: A Review of the Links. Diabetes Spectrum, 18(2), 121-127.

How I survived 40 years with diabetes

www.ingramcontent.com/pod-product-compliance
Lightning Source LLC
Chambersburg PA
CBHW070950220526
45471CB00007B/2969